I Had Two
When
I Came In

I Had Two When I Came In

Ellie Wyatt

Library of Congress Control Number: 2011915585
ISBN: Hardcover   978-1-4653-6044-1
                 Softcover   978-1-4653-6043-4
                 Ebook   978-1-4653-6045-8

To order additional copies of this book, contact:
Xlibris Corporation
1-888-795-4274
www.Xlibris.com
Orders@Xlibris.com
102242

To my husband
Who never screamed at the sight
Of the lopsided vision
Of one left on the right.

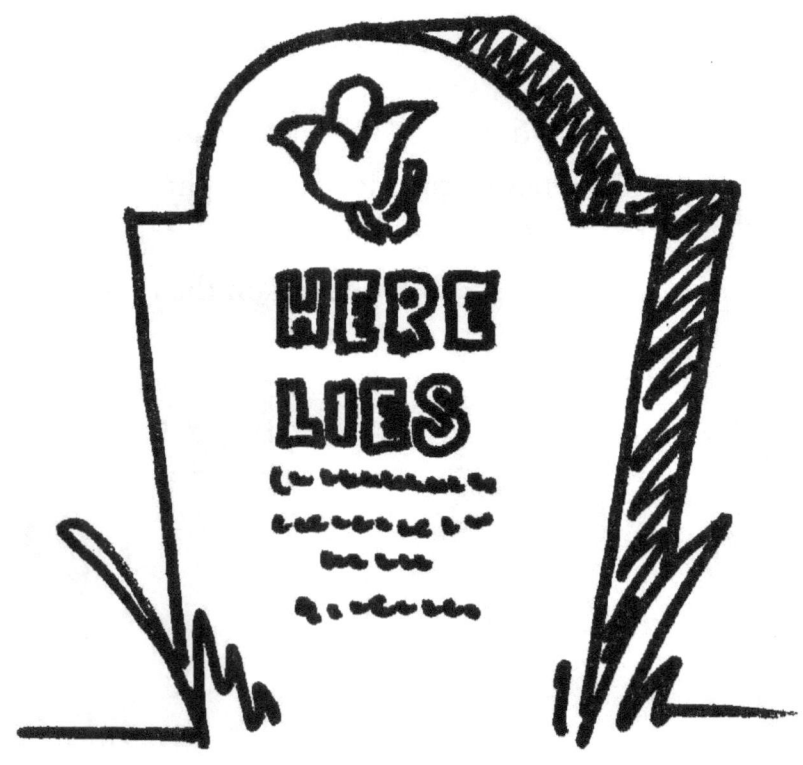

Mastectomy is no joke at all
But if this is the category in which you fall
You're better off to have one side flat
Than to rest on a slab—flat on your back.

ELLIE WYATT

PREFACE

T HE TITLE OF this book was chosen for two reasons. First, it's an attention getter and the subject it covers needs attention. Second, it's a true story—the story of my battle with breast cancer. No matter how grim and traumatic the experience is for any woman, I must remark somewhat facetiously that, in one respect, the title is misleading. Prior to the operation, I was not one of those females who had been richly endowed by nature. So perhaps a more fitting title would be *I Had Too Little When I Came In*. It follows that even though I lost one, I cannot claim the loss was overwhelmingly large.

My purpose in relating the story of my mastectomy and subsequent metastatic disease is rooted in the hope that the telling will help educate women in what to expect if they should become breast cancer patients. If I can reach just one and pull her fears from the darkness that comes from lack of knowledge and information, I will have achieved that purpose. I wish someone had informed me.

Some women have a continuing and gnawing fear of malignancy of the breast. I never had such fear. It was something that suddenly afflicted other people, not me. Possibly, I even thought a lump couldn't grow in the small area I could furnish. As a matter of fact, in my entire life, I never had a conversation on the subject with anyone. Of course, I knew of several women who had had breasts removed, but it was a deep, dark secret, nothing to be talked about. I refuse to accept the hush-hush attitude. It isn't healthy and helps no one who needs help after the doctor has said, "Cancer!"

The innumerable books and articles written on the subject by doctors, surgeons, psychiatrists, and other specialists are erudite and filled with medical terms that mean little to the layman. They merely convey what the learned medicos have absorbed from observation and study. A woman facing reality of the fearful fact needs more than that. She needs, as they say in the vernacular, someone to tell it like it is.

Thus, in this account, I offer no high-flown technical or medical phraseology. I just tell it like it is.

I 'M FORTY-FIVE YEARS old and married. I've had three children. I've worked twenty-seven years in the secretarial and court-reporting fields.

About three years ago, I began losing quite a bit of time from work—a day off here and a day off there. I wasn't feeling really well. Coworkers urged me to get a complete medical checkup. I had noticed a lump in my breast. I knew many women have cysts or lumps from the menstrual cycle. I felt sure the lump would go away, but it didn't.

One Sunday evening, I felt really ill. Even my children were surprised when I went to bed without eating dinner. They weren't accustomed to seeing Mother in a horizontal position that early in the evening. I've always had an aversion to going to bed early. I think it's a waste of time to sleep unless you're really tired.

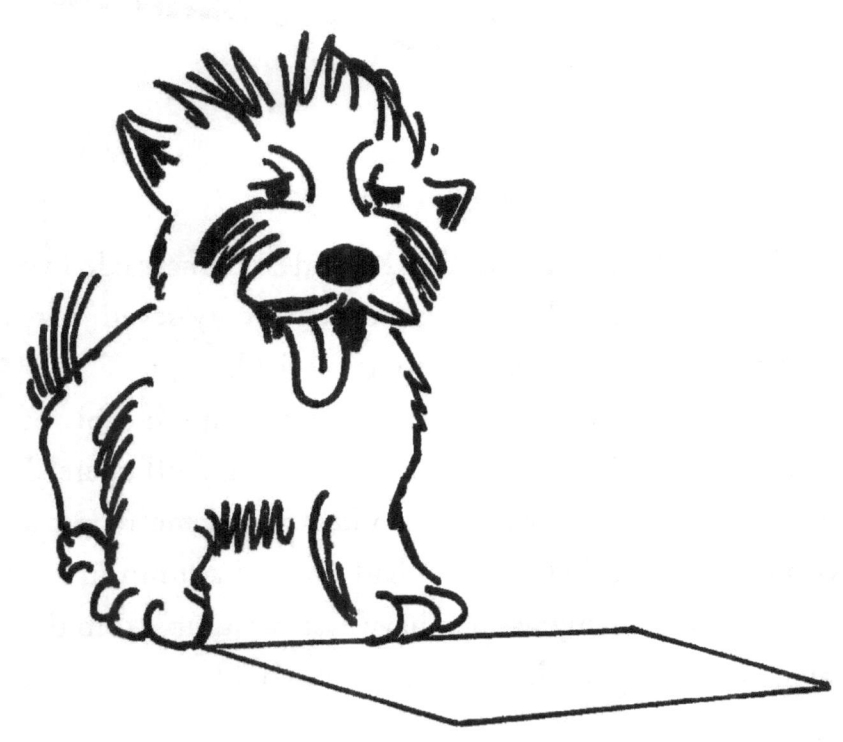

Losing a breast need not blur your reason
Or make you a dropout during mating season.

ELLIE WYATT

The next day, I gave in and went to the doctor for a checkup. During the examination, the lump was checked, and the usual oohs and ahs began. The doctor immediately sent me to a surgeon. When the word *cancer* came from him, I was astounded. No, that isn't the word. It was like walking into a strange big dark room with no light switch to flip. I had no idea what to expect. And I was scared, sick scared. Cancer just couldn't be happening to me.

I thought of my three youngsters, my husband, our home. I knew—and the knowledge came like a flash of lightning—I was needed. I had a responsibility to live. I couldn't fall apart in despair. I resolved then and there to accept my responsibility as I had never before accepted it. As long as I had breath, I would fight. With God's help, I would do everything I could.

I resolved several other things that day. In my uphill battle—win, lose, or draw—I would neither lament nor bemoan my misfortune. Life for my family would be as normal as the Good Lord would allow me to make it. If need be, I would laugh, sing, go through the daily routines with some semblance of gaiety. Most importantly, I would reacquire my failing sense of humor. In short, if in the end I had to go down, I would do it with courage and banners flying. These resolutions were the best of my life. Coupled with my faith, they have made these *living* years ones in which my appreciations and perceptions have sharpened and matured.

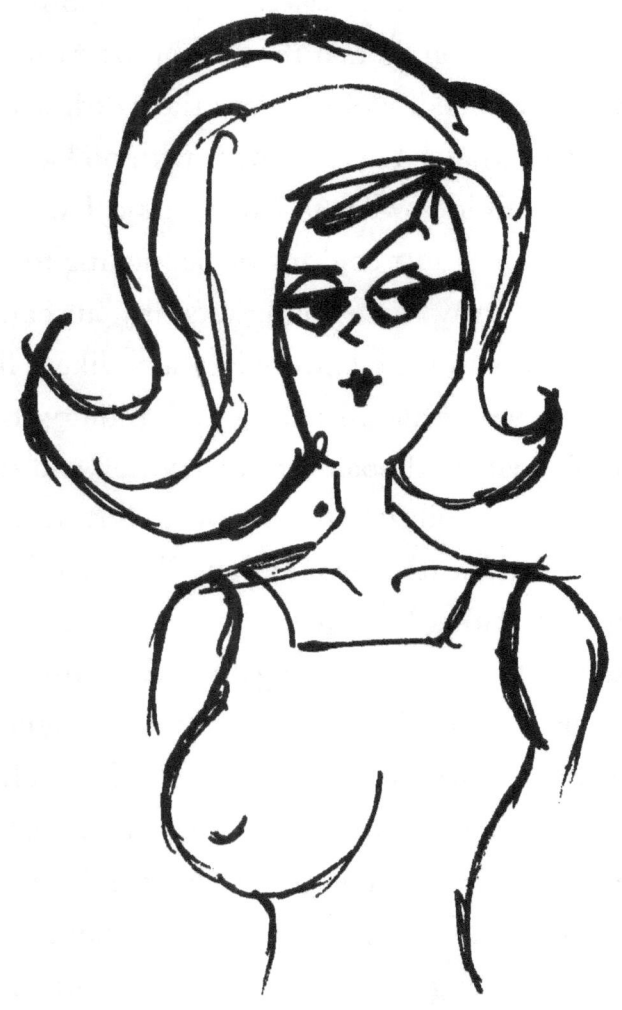

You certainly learn where it's really at—
When you wake up in recovery—and one side's flat.

ELLIE WYATT

If I hadn't had faith that all would be well—in time—I don't think I could have undergone the various phases of treatments that have taken place to date. My lack of knowledge was frightening. I soon learned that getting information was not easy. I'm not really a religious person, but I do have faith. There's a difference between being religious and having faith.

On April 13, 1971, a radical mastectomy (complete breast removal) was performed. I was in a large hospital. The biopsy was taken while I was in surgery and sedated. It was immediately tested in the pathology lab of the hospital. It was found to be malignant, and the breast was removed immediately. Prior to entering the hospital, I had to sign a document giving permission to remove the breast if malignancy was found. After the biopsy, my doctor informed my husband of the results (in the waiting room) and told him what would be done.

I can't elaborate on my emotions immediately following the mastectomy. It was a long operation. I recall vaguely being half awake. I had gone to the operating room about 9:30 a.m. When I awakened, I remember looking at the clock in my room. It was 7:00 p.m. and dark outside. My husband was standing by my bed. Everything was blurry.

I asked weakly, "Did they take it off?"

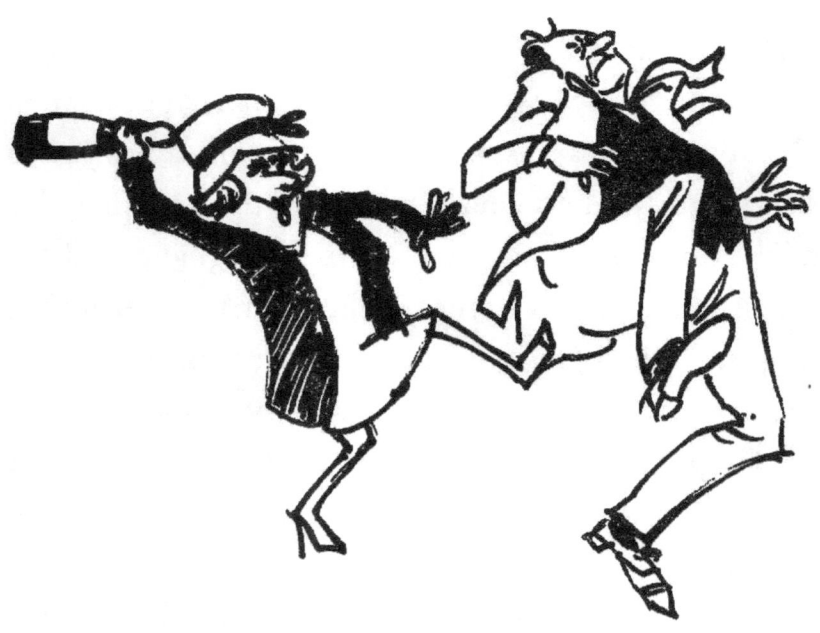

If you're wondering if your mate will stammer and shudder
Over absence of one, or maybe the udder,
Don't let it depress you or get you uptight
If he can't accept it, get him way out of sight.

ELLIE WYATT

I saw him simply nod his head. I slipped back into a deep sleep that lasted until the next morning.

It's important to remember that there should be close coordination between a mastectomy patient, her surgeon, and the anesthesiologist. I have always been a deep-sleep individual. After my long mastectomy, the nurses in the recovery room had difficulty awakening me. As a result of my experience, I think the anesthesiologist should personally see all mastectomy patients and discuss their possible reactions to sleep-inducing medications.

On April 20, a week after the removal of my breast, further major surgery was performed to remove my ovaries. This is called an oophorectomy. My doctor's treatment for breast cancer includes removal of the ovaries in order to bring on change of life and stop the menstrual period. He explained that removal precludes possibility of the hormones running rampant through the body during the menstrual cycle. Hormones are believed by some scientists to contribute to the cancer's potential. I also had taken the birth control pill for three years, between the births of my second and third child. Whether or not birth control pills are a contributing factor in cancer still is up in the medical air.

Personally, the only effect I noticed while taking the pill was jangled nerves. I would rant and rave over trivial things, and this was not my usual behavior. Also, I never

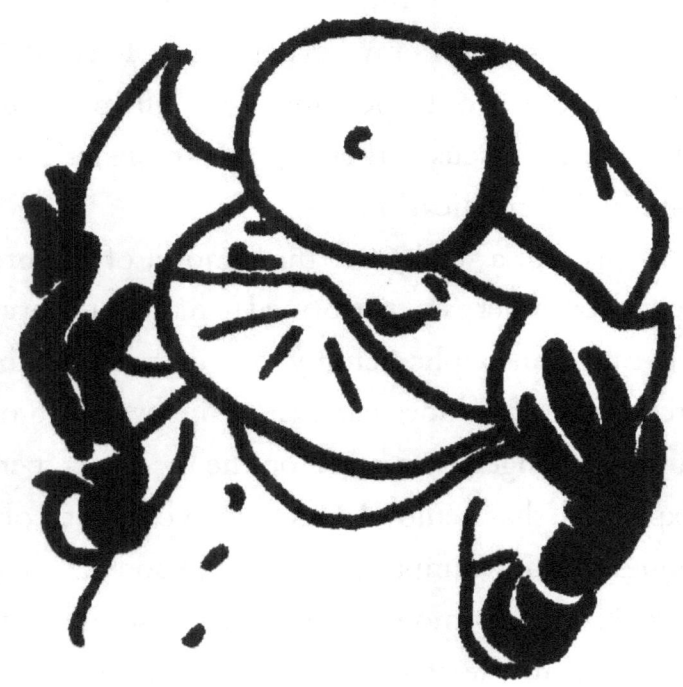

No one knows during life's short tour
What will befall them, that's for sure.
But we who undergo the knife for cancer
Are helping science to find the answer.

ELLIE WYATT

had had headaches until I took the pill. Those ceased when I decided to eliminate it.

I went home on April 25. On April 28, I was scheduled to begin daily morning cobalt treatments at the medical center downtown. This required my driving to and from the treatment center five days each week for almost six weeks (about ten miles each way). My husband and friends offered to drive me, but if my husband took time off to serve as chauffeur, it would have meant shorter paychecks for him. With all the doctor's bills, I couldn't let him do that. My friends were sincere in their offers too, but I felt it would be an imposition. Besides, I felt I was capable of driving.

Actually, I never stayed in bed after I got home from the hospital, except of course for my regular night's sleep. This was not too wise. I was run-down, lost more weight, and felt terribly weak and depressed. Adequate rest probably would have prevented these complications.

The first time I reported for cobalt treatment, I was ushered into an enormous sealed room. The monstrous cobalt 60 machine stood in the center. I was instructed to strip from the waist up and lie on the table part of the machine. The attendant adjusted the machinery to my body, marking Xs to denote treatment spots, then left the room. She closed the big door and turned on the cobalt from a control point outside. There was a small window

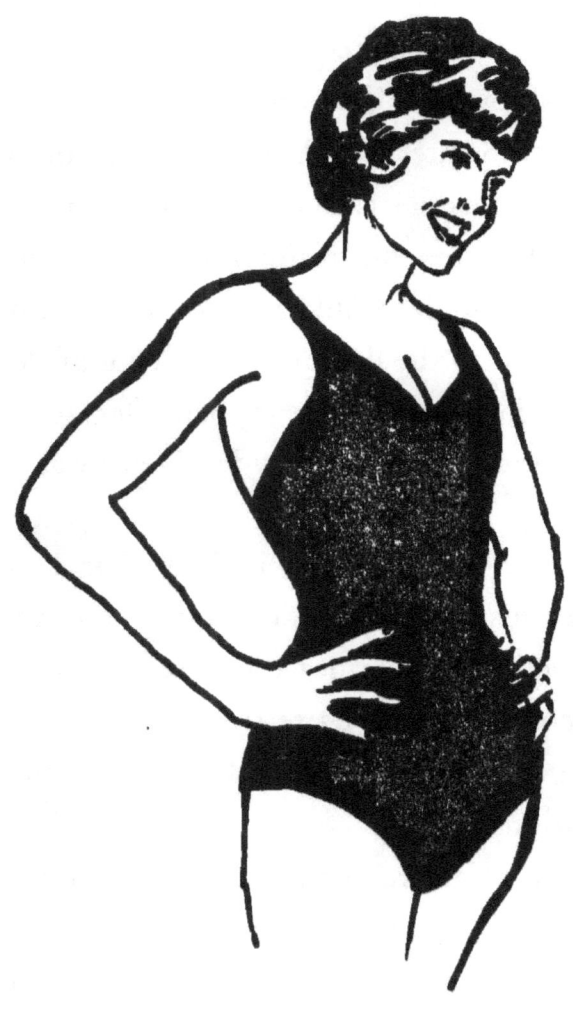

What is left may not be wriggly,
But you can become understudy to Twiggy.

ELLIE WYATT

where she could watch me. The machine itself is frightening. Also, I hardly knew what to expect—whether the treatment would hurt or how it would affect me. That day, I inquired if there was any literature I could read or which they would furnish so I could familiarize myself with the treatment and possible side effects of the cobalt. I was told I would be informed of anything that I had to know.

After the second week of treatment, I became charred like a piece of charcoal all over the front half of my body, from waist to neck as well as on my back, but the pain was no more than that of a severe sunburn but was very uncomfortable. I had to wear a certain type of clothing to cover the burned skin. The attendant told me they had never seen anyone burn as severely as me. The only information I received was a warning that I might become nauseous after treatments, but that never happened. When the burn set in, itching began day and night. It was impossible to sleep or do anything else. About six weeks later, the burning stopped, but the itching didn't. I scratched ceaselessly and frantically. Finally, I insisted my doctor do something to relieve the itching. He prescribed an ointment that made the itching bearable, so at least, I could get some sleep.

When the itching began to subside, the cobalt, causing drying of the lung tissues, brought on a very bad cough. This persisted day and night. There

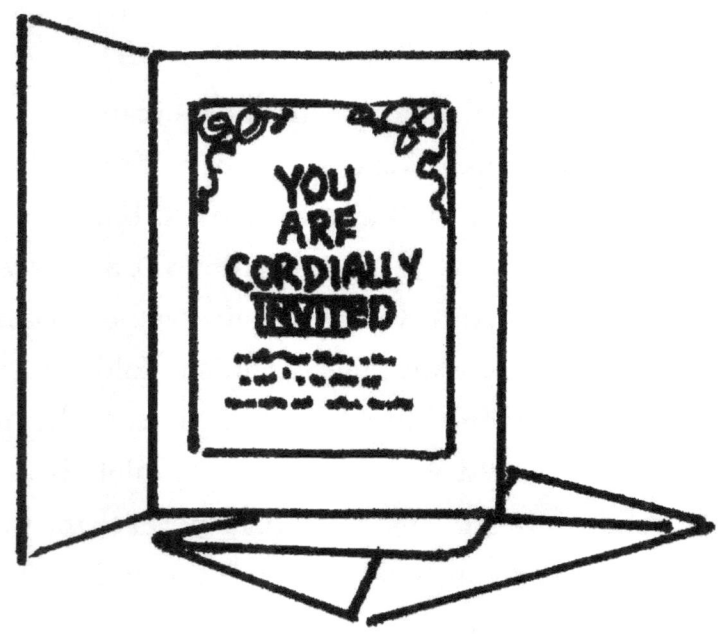

They say curiosity killed the cat,

But satisfaction brought it back.

If people are curious to see your operation,

Tell them it requires an engraved invitation.

ELLIE WYATT

wasn't too much I could do for the cough. I am unable to take any kind of medication that induces sleep or drowsiness. I can hardly take a glass of anything containing even alcohol without almost passing out. Perhaps the cough would not have been as severe for a nonsmoker. I feel sure, however, that drying of the lung tissues induces violent coughing whether you smoke or not.

Within two weeks after the oophorectomy, the usual symptoms of menopause began—namely, hot flashes, heavy perspiration, blurred vision, and extreme discomfort. Any woman who has undergone menopause is familiar with this. In most instances, doctors can administer estrogen hormones to alleviate the menopausal symptoms. That was my hope too until I questioned my doctor. He told me he could not give me anything to help since hormones may further cancer development. I just had to live with it. During the period of "living through" the side effects of cobalt, the menopausal symptoms made my life not only uncomfortable but miserable as well. I know now that side effects from cobalt extend over a four—to six-month period. Of course, no one told me this. I had to experience it.

I had one good side effect from cobalt. It burned off the underarm hair on the side being treated. The hair just seemed to disappear. Now I only have to shave under one arm. It's a good thing too because it's numb under the

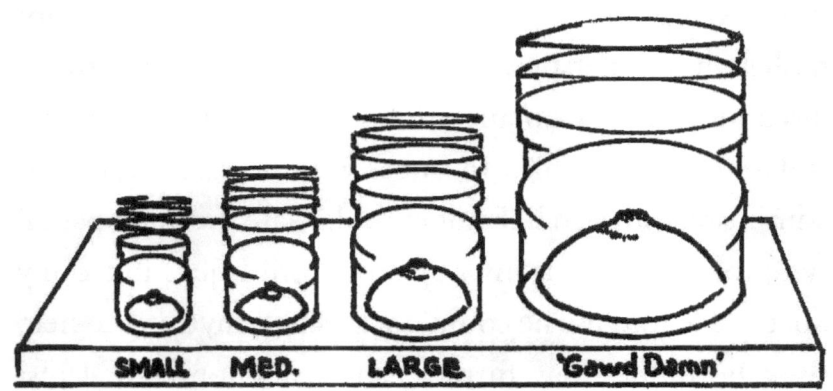

Wonder what becomes of those they take off
The round, the firm, the pretty and soft.
Maybe they're shelved in a room in seclusion,
And completing the picture of my illusion
Labeled small, large, or from medium-frame
But never known by their once-owners' name.

ELLIE WYATT

arm of my "treated" side, and I'd probably cut myself every time I used a razor.

A number of women I met at the cobalt center were taking the same treatment for breast cancer. I noticed that all those I met had difficulty in moving their arms. In a radical mastectomy, the lymph nodes are cut on the underarm of the affected side to ascertain whether the glands also are cancerous. Luckily, mine were not. I never had any difficulty raising my arm. I recall that the morning after my breast was removed, my surgeon came in to see me. The first thing he did was ask if I could raise my arm. I put it right up over my head just as I had always done. He seemed amazed. I'm left-handed, and it was the left arm. I can't say whether it would have been this way if the operation had been performed on my right arm. Actually, the only limitation I've noticed in that arm is weakness when I try to open a tight jar lid or pick up a heavy object. If there is difficulty moving the affected arm, exercise will help.

The prosthesis is a major part of a breast cancer patient's rehabilitation. It is necessary for balance. Also, it helps a woman regain confidence, makes clothes fit properly, and helps make her look just as she always did.

The prosthesis fitting should be arranged as soon as possible after the mastectomy. I was wearing my prosthesis within four weeks after surgery. Usually, the soreness is gone by then.

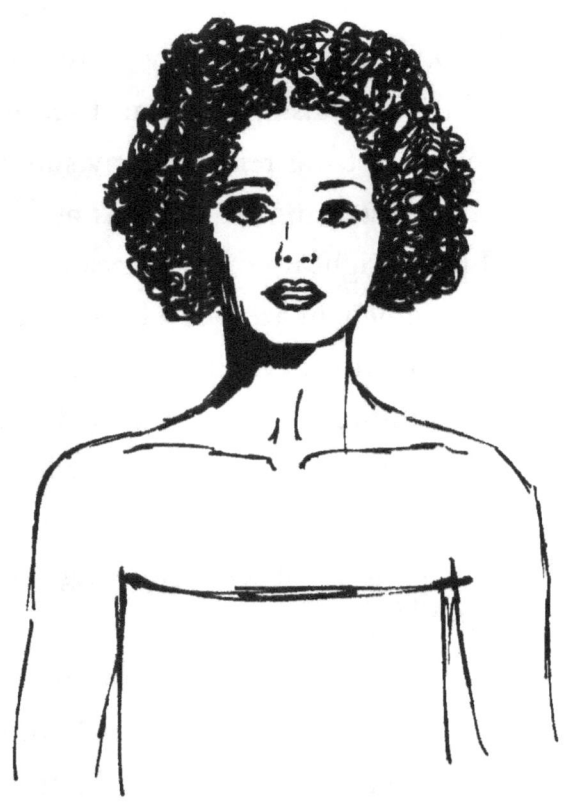

A hefty bosom was once the female goal,
But modern emphasis calls for soul.

ELLIE WYATT

As of now, there are three types of prosthesis. I believe the type I chose is, by far, the best. It is the most expensive but will cost less over the years. It is made of silicone. It looks and feels almost like the real thing. In fact, it even acquires your body temperature while being worn. If it is punctured, it even reseals itself. It can be worn inside any normal bra. Also, it can be cleansed with mild soap and warm water as many times a day as you like. After wearing mine for three years, it's just like new.

The other two types, in my opinion, are not as serviceable, but some women might prefer them because of the lower initial cost. One is foam filled and is an insert. It must be worn with a special bra made just for the insert. The third type is an insert filled with liquid and must also be worn with a special bra. If punctured with a corsage pin, it would be ruined—and the leakage could cause embarrassment. Although the foam and liquid-filled insert types are less expensive, cost of the special bra must be taken into consideration. With this information, you should be well filled-in.

I returned to work during the fourth week of my cobalt treatments by arranging a change in the treatment time to coincide with my working hours. I knew the sooner I returned to work, the better I would feel and the less chance I would have to start feeling sorry for myself. I was already at the stage when every time I saw a woman flaunting her bosom on television, I would cry.

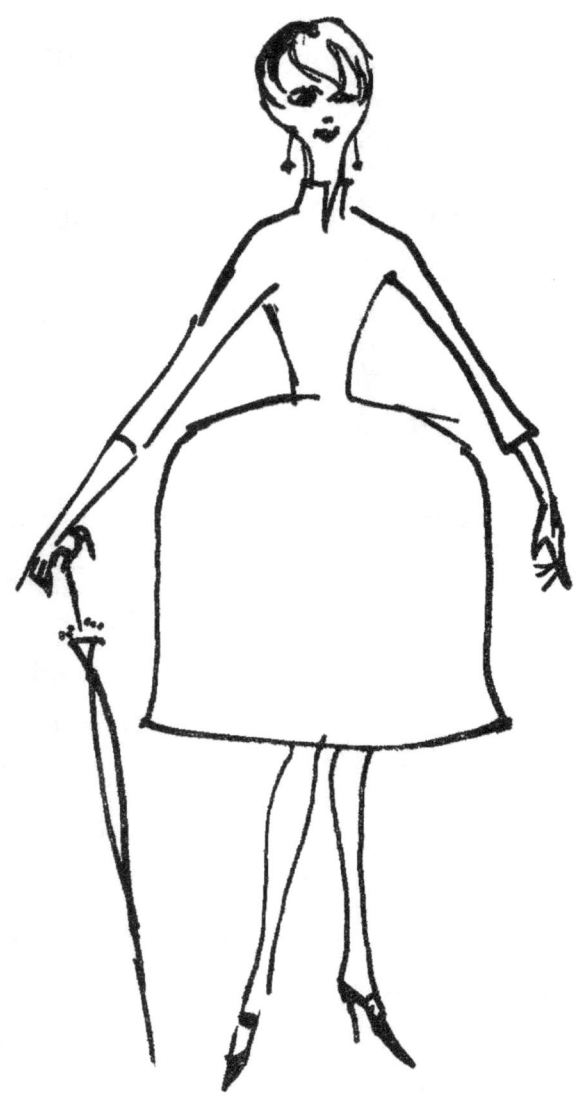

So one is gone and loudly lamented,
But that's no reason to become demented.
Rise and shine and make your plans
For a brand-new you as fast as you can.

ELLIE WYATT

I felt fine. I was so glad to be alive and back to my regular routine. I was under the impression that the only thing I had to worry about was the possibility of the cancer spreading to the other breast. This was May in 1971. My youngest child was four years old. My most fervent hope is to see him grow up.

In September, I signed up for a refresher course for secretaries. A month later, I passed a test and was certified in shorthand (taken by hand) at 140 words per minute. That really encouraged me. Also, on August 1, 1971, I had received a merit promotion.

But by the end of November, I began having severe neck pains in the cervical spine area. The longer I sat at my desk, the worse the pain grew. I kept mentioning this to my doctor at each checkup period. He prescribed nerve pills and tranquilizers, advising me against working so hard. Of course, I didn't have any of the prescriptions filled since I knew they would only make me ill. The pain persisted. Finally, in March of 1972, I insisted that my doctor try to determine what was causing the pain. Tests were run. The cancer had gone to the spine, with deterioration of the bone, or metastatic disease.

I will try to convey my reactions when I received the news of the metastatic disease. I became quite emotional. For a few hours, I was totally grief stricken and at a loss. I didn't know how I could go on. I pictured myself

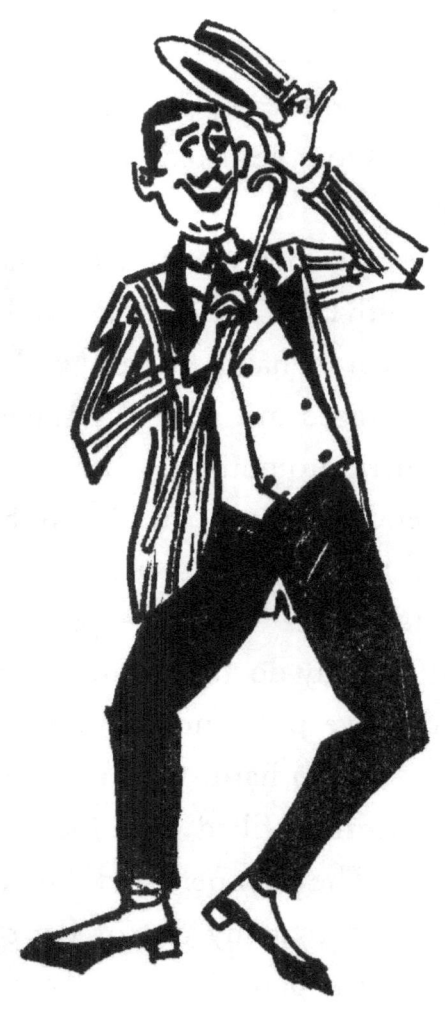

A prosthesis to replace what you've lost
Is worth every penny of the cost.
With it you can win the bets they make
On which one's real and which one's fake.

ELLIE WYATT

deteriorating rapidly. After the tests, I had been told I would be informed of the results. My doctor's nurse called me at work on a Friday afternoon and said the doctor wanted to see me. This was unusual and frightening. Early the next morning, he handed me the written report, saying he could hardly believe this had happened after the extensive preventive treatment I had undergone.

That particular Saturday was a rough day for me. I finally pulled myself together, looked at my children, and came to my senses. I fell back on my faith after a few hours of self-pity.

News of the malignancy of the lump in the breast was not nearly as shaking as the report of metastatic disease. Perhaps the reason for that is I knew the lump was there. I could feel it. It was real. There were only two questions—malignant or benign?

The spinal pain was different. When it began, I thought the worst it could be was arthritis. Of course, you do hope a lump in the breast is benign, but it can be accepted more readily than a spread of the cancer. For those few tear-filled hours on that Saturday, I could think of nothing but dying and dreading the crippling stages I might suffer first. Now here I am two years later. Although I'm retired from my secretarial work, I can still move my fingers well enough to type this book. I attribute this to faith that followed total despair.

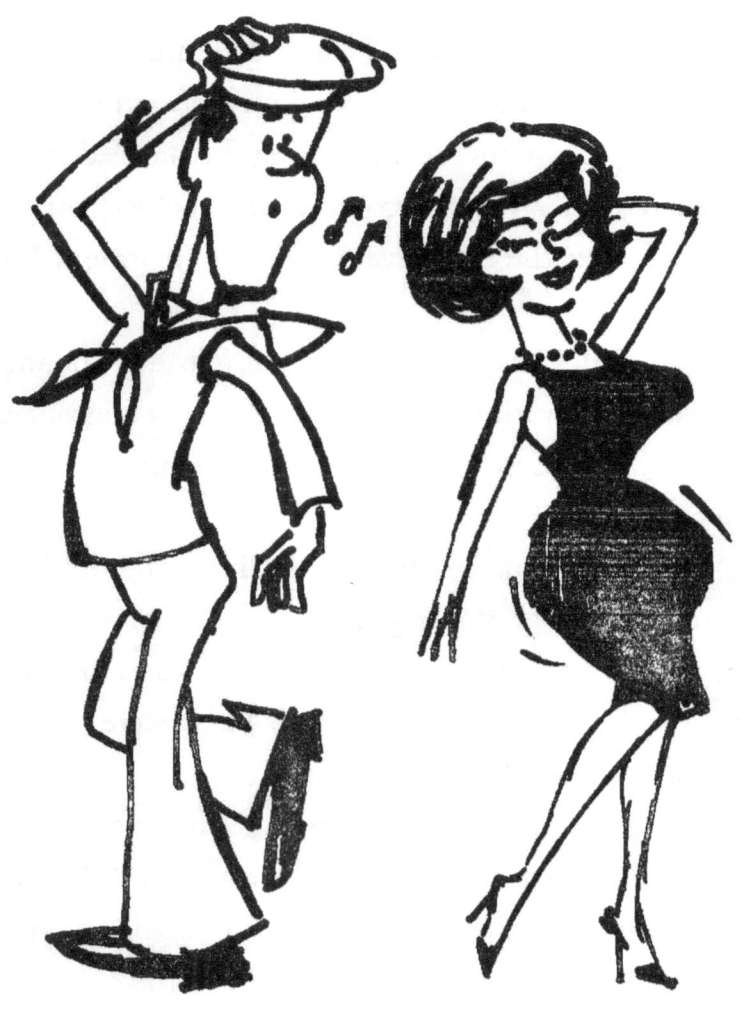

The prosthesis is a marvelous invention
Comes in any size which can be mentioned
So if you didn't have so much to lose,
Your new bustline can be any size you choose.

ELLIE WYATT

After the diagnosis of metastatic disease, there were more tests done by an orthopedic doctor, a neurosurgeon, a rehabilitation specialist, and an internal medicine specialist. The chemotherapist then took over as my principal doctor. The metastatic disease is controlled with male hormones taken in pill form. The male hormones counteract the female hormones. They also ease the pain and make it bearable. The only side effects I have noted from male hormones are more hair growth and deepening of my heretofore feminine voice.

After the diagnosis, when sitting at a desk all day was becoming increasingly difficult, the doctors advised me to retire. I did—in June of 1972. The adjustment of suddenly being "just a housewife" after so many years of working was a big step for me.

I know that much time and effort have been devoted to the somber, serious side of breast cancer on shows like *Medical Center, Marcus Welby*, and others. That's fine. But the fact that there are so many mastectomy patients still around and very much alive warrants a lighter side to the subject, a tribute to us, and a salute to the prosthesis. Thanks to the prosthesis industry, I, for one, look like the same old person.

But don't let me or anyone else tell you the trauma that results from a mastectomy won't bring about a good many psychic reactions. You're changed. You're different. There have been physical changes. While a woman is

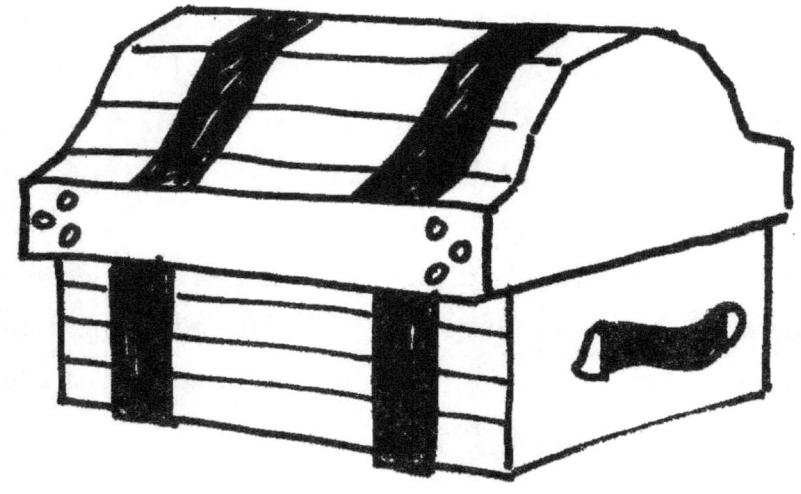

There is a word that rhymes with *city*
The chesty subject of this little ditty,
But mammary gland might be better taste
Particularly since it's gone to waste.
But the choicest word behind that lump
Can be placed with it in the city dump.
It served you long and probably well,
But it had to go—so what the hell!

ELLIE WYATT

pregnant, for example, she feels clumsy, awkward, unattractive, and unloved. After the baby is born, she feels beautiful again. Mastectomy, on the other hand, is permanent. A main part of your femininity is gone. Some women have the impression that a silicone operation can restore the breast. That's not so if you have a mastectomy. You need tissue for a silicone operation. In a radical mastectomy, all tissue is removed.

If you're married, you'll go through periods of feeling that there is no way your husband can still love you. You'll hate every woman who has her feminine charms intact. If you're a single woman, you'll vow no man could ever look at you. These are normal reactions. Time, faith, and a sense of humor can conquer them.

Mastectomy separates the girls from the women. You can be a girl with a deep-rooted sense of shallow vanity, or you can be a woman who can maintain pride and dignity under any circumstances. False pride shows up much easier than a false breast.

Women definitely need to establish healthy attitudes toward breast cancer. It can happen to any woman. Face it and learn all you can. Demand to know. Some women say they would never have a breast removed. When and if it ever comes to the decision, what would you do? I don't doubt you would do the same as I.

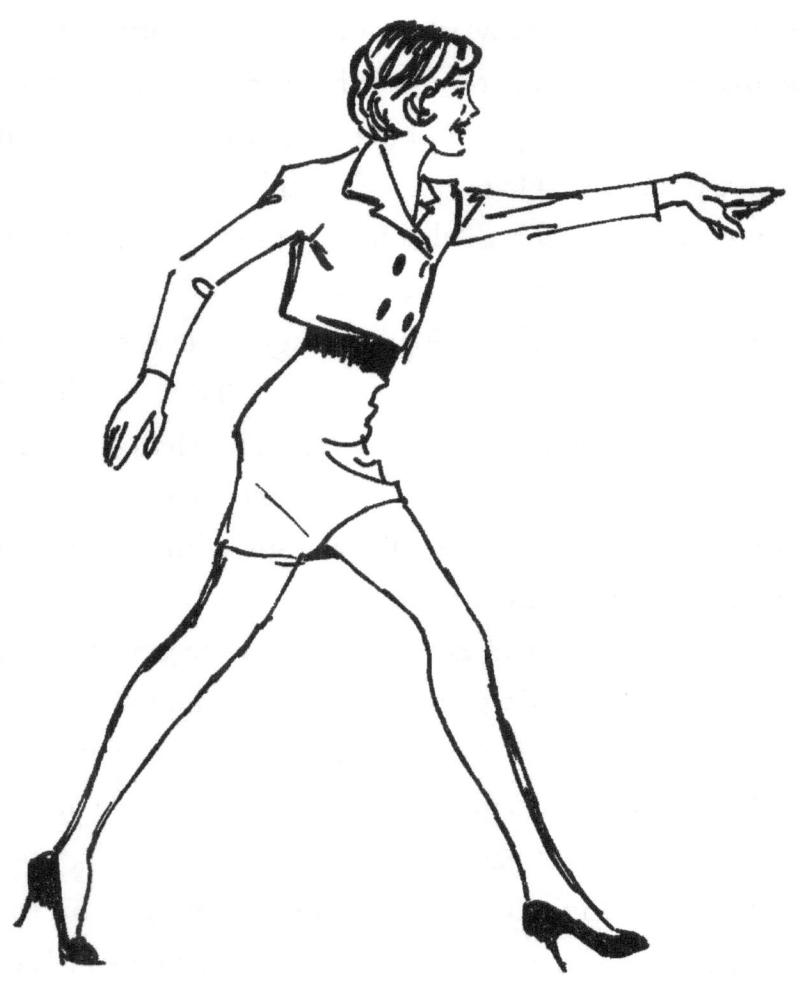

A light-sided view I herein impart,
On a subject so dear to my heart.
To urge mastectomy patients to always thrive
In a thought like mine—I'm still alive.

ELLIE WYATT

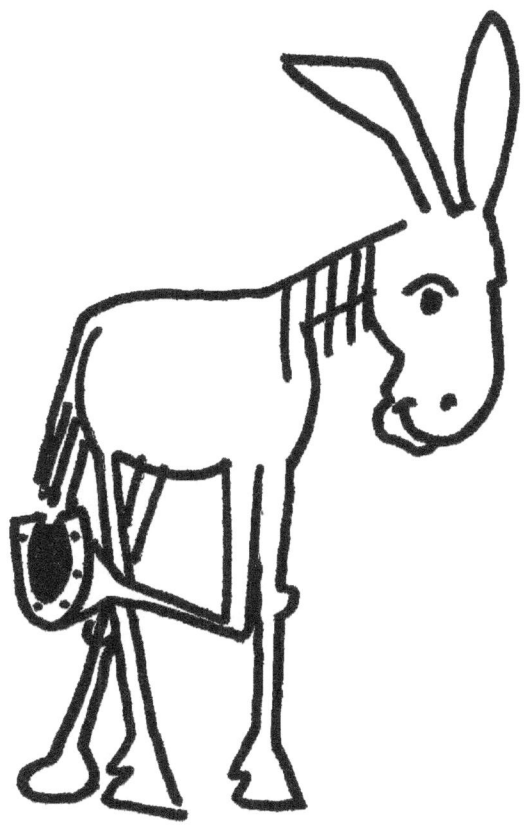

If they take your breastworks, my dear,
You still can flaunt what makes up your rear.

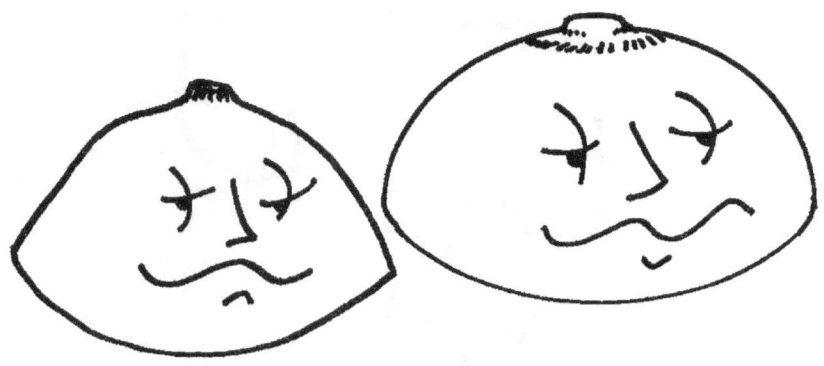

Whether stuffed with special foam
Or a prosthesis made of silicone,
A breast by any thought-up name
Somehow really feels the same.

ELLIE WYATT

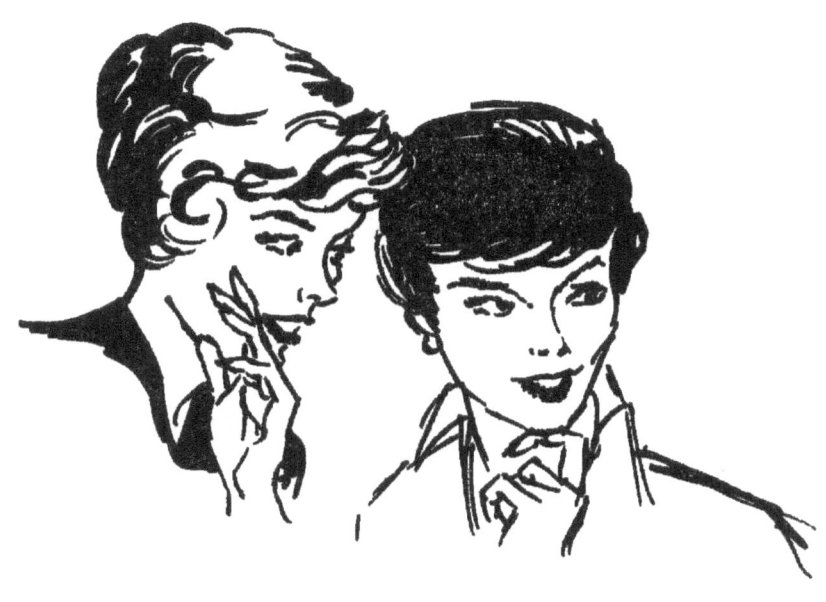

When they yack about your loss of breast,
Laugh it off—it's a load off your chest.

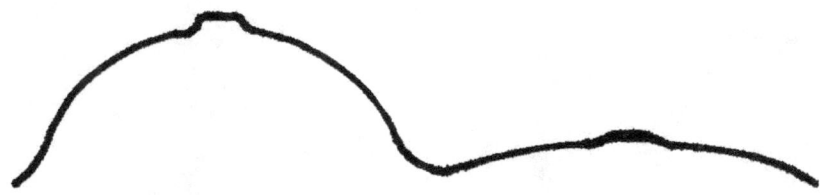

I had two when I came in, I know,
Then the surgeon said the lump must go.
While I was sedated and very still,
From a mountain he made a small molehill.

　　　　　　　　　ELLIE WYATT

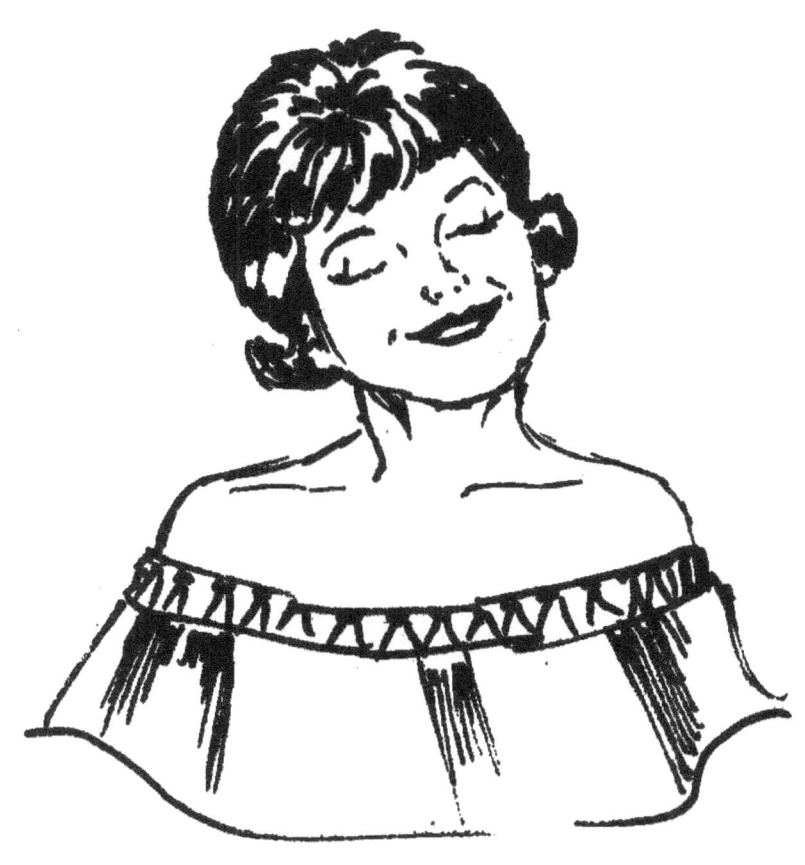

Medical science has helped us greatly, dears.

Half our chests are gone but we are here.

Going for broke in life's big whirl

Doesn't require appendages of a go-go girl!

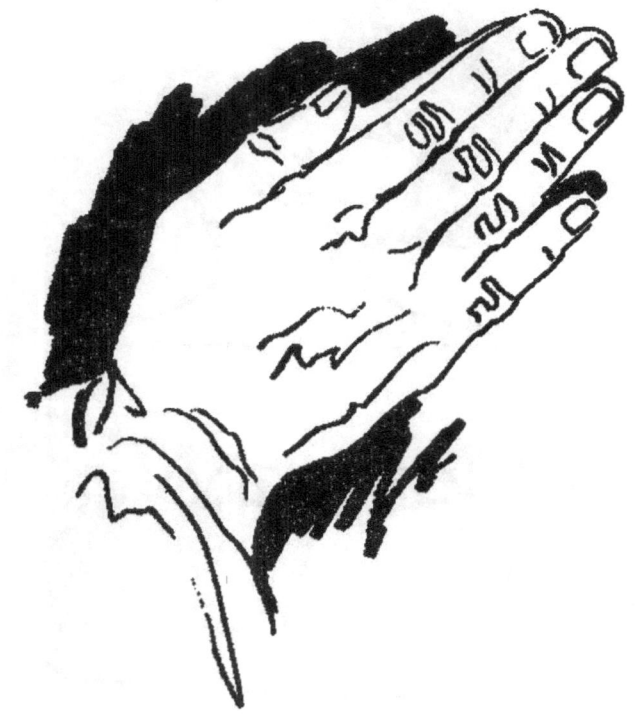

True, undaunted faith and a keen sense of humor
Can carry you through an ordeal with a tumor.
Only with heart and soul is the adjustment real,
If your faith is like mine, then you know how I feel.

ELLIE WYATT

*F*ASCINATING, VERY CREATIVE. *Congratulations to this great lady of courage and determination!*

—Elizabeth Lancaster, executive director
Hillsborough County Unit
American Cancer Society

I Had Two When I Came In *is one woman's confrontation with cancer of the breast. It reveals a very personal experience that is shared by many and dreaded by all women. Not all women with breast cancer will receive the same treatment given Ellie Wyatt, but most will be subjected to the same emotional and psychological stresses associated with removal of the breast. Her success in adjusting to the realities of cancer and to her new body image is evident throughout. The book, written with courage and humor, is Mrs. Wyatt's gift to any who may face the same disease with its medical consequences.*

—David M. Richter, MD, Major, USAF
Chief, General Surgery
MacDill AFB Hospital

ABOUT THE AUTHOR

ELLIE WYATT CAME through the mastectomy operation beautifully. It was her lack of information that made her suffer the most. She became determined she would do everything in her power to help prevent other women from going through the same experience she did—no information when faced with cancer.

Her account of the different phases of treatment she underwent for breast cancer is extremely informative. The satirical slant is refreshingly presented.

Ellie Wyatt is one of a pair of identical twins, and as she points out, her twin sister is still "all together." They both were the last of a family of fifteen children raised in Woodside, Long Island, New York.

When she was twenty-four, Ellie Wyatt joined the US Air Force during the Korean conflict. During the time she spent in the air force, she became a court reporter. After being honorably discharged from the air force, she went into legal secretarial work. She's been recording secretary on the executive board of Local Union 173 of the International Brotherhood of Teamsters, publicity chairman of the Key West Chapter of the National Association of Legal Secretaries, has been a notary public since 1955, worked in income tax at Wards and Sears, and completed approximately ten years in federal civil service. She also writes poetry, which she would like to see transformed into music.

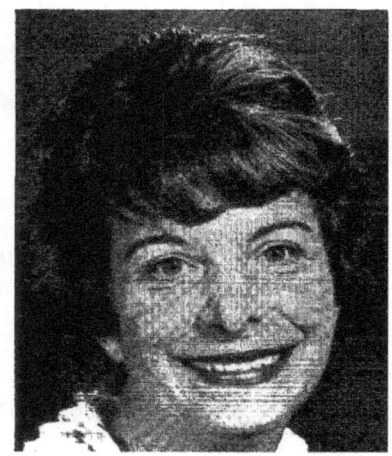

Ellie Wyatt

During her working career of twenty-seven years, Ellie took a three-year correspondence course in journalism from Palmers Writers School. She's also married and has three children aged seven, twelve, and seventeen. As she says, they were born on the five-year warranty plan. Her husband, Fred, is employed by Pan American Aerospace Division as a range station technician.

The title of her book in itself, *I Had Two When I Came In*, is indicative of Ellie Wyatt's sense of gallows humor and satyr. Her chief goals are informing women and helping cancer victims achieve a better outlook on their new lifestyle.